No More Yeast Infection

The Complete Guide on Yeast Infection
Symptoms, Causes, Treatments & A
Holistic Approach to Cure Yeast
Infection, Eliminate Candida, Naturally
& Permanently

Julie J. Stone
Copyright© 2014 by Julie J. Stone

No More Yeast Infection

Copyright© 2014 Julie J. Stone

Publisher: Living Plus Healthy Publishing

ISBN-13: 978-1497453029

ISBN-10: 149745302X

Disclaimer

The Publisher has strived to be as accurate and complete as possible in the creation of this book. While all attempts have been made to verify information provided in this publication, the Publisher assumes no responsibility for errors, omissions, or contrary interpretation of the subject matter herein. Any perceived slights of specific persons, peoples, or organizations are unintentional.

This book is not intended for use as a source of legal, business, accounting or financial advice. All readers are advised to seek services of competent professionals in the legal, business, accounting, and finance fields.

The information in this book is not intended or implied to be a substitute for professional medical advice, diagnosis or treatment. All content contained in this book is for general information purposes only. Always consult your healthcare provider before carrying on any health program.

Table of Contents

Introduction

Nearly every woman will experience a yeast infection in her life. The burning and stinging on her vaginal skin is typically accompanied by a foul-smelling white discharge that is particularly embarrassing to endure and seek help for.

However, women are certainly not the only people who get yeast infections. Everyone—men, women, children, babies and the elderly are all at risk. Yeast infections are caused by Candida, a micro-organism that naturally lives in the body. While it is typically harmless, an imbalance can cause it to grow out of control, overtake the bacteria that usually keep it in check and cause a multitude of symptoms.

While women are known to suffer from vaginal yeast infections, the Candida can also affect men's genitalia (most often by having sexual intercourse with a woman infected with a yeast infection).

An overgrowth of yeast can occur any-where on the body: In the mouth, it creates an unsightly white coating or small bumps. On the finger or toenails, it can cause the nail to crumple, lift from the nail bed and even fall off.

It is often confused with jock itch in men (which is caused by a different sort of fungus) and yeast can feel right at home anywhere the skin folds and creates a warm, moist breeding ground for the yeast. This typically happens under the breasts, in the armpits or under the scrotum. For those who are overweight, yeast can run rampant in the folds of excess skin.

At its worst, a yeast infection that festers in the intestines can eat through the stomach lin-ing and cause a blood infection. This is a seri-ous and potentially life-threatening circum-stance.

As horrible as yeast infections are, diag-nosing them and getting the yeast under con-trol is typically quick and inexpensive with medication, particularly if caught in the early stages. For those who have recurring yeast in-fections, more serious diet and lifestyle chang-es need to be adhered to. Some people— especially those with weak immune systems or diseases like AIDS or cancer—will need to make dramatic changes to their diets, that include detoxing and maintaining a healthier body overall.

This book delves into all of the causes for yeast infections in various body parts as well as traditional medical intervention, home remedies and diet changes that can cure you of your yeast infection once and for all and relieve those unpleasant symptoms. You may need your doctor at first to help you control the infection, but then you should be able to take your health into your own hands and keep yeast out of your life.

Chapter 1: What is Yeast Infection?

Living inside your body are millions of micro-organisms. Most of these are harmless and live in harmony with one another in a delicate balance. One of these micro-organisms is Candida, which is normally found in the human body. There are more than 20 types of Candida, and it usually lives among other flora without incident.

However, when the balance of the micro-organisms goes out of whack, Candida can turn into a pathogen, a dangerous infectious agent that creates unfavorable outcomes for your health. This imbalance causes Candida to multiply quickly in a fungus form.

The most common type is *Candida albicans*, which develops into the white, cheesy like yeast that is found typically in areas where the skin is moist (the mouth, underarms and vagina, most notably). Babies are particularly susceptible to yeast infections in their mouths as well as when wearing wet diapers. This uncomfortable condition causes severe itching and burning on the skin.

This overgrowth of Candida is known as *candidiasis* and occurs when there are not enough friendly flora bacteria to keep the Candida levels in check or when the skin cannot block out yeast growth because of an injury to the skin which allows the yeast to find its way in. This ongoing battle can weaken the body's immunity and lead to a number of symptoms.

When the yeast overwhelms the other bacteria, it can infect on a surface level, such as the skin, but left unchecked, it can grow throughout your entire body—even in your blood stream. While seemingly superficial infections may appear simply bothersome, deeper infections can lead to serious health issues, such as leaky gut syndrome, which is when the yeast grows through the intestinal wall and allows undigested food and the yeast to enter the blood stream. In some cases, a burrowing yeast infection can be life-threatening.

Not Only Women Are In Danger

Many people think of yeast infections as being something only women suffer from; and it is true that about 70 percent of cases are females (since Candida causes estrogen levels to dip so that progesterone levels will increase—and Candida likes to feed off of progesterone.)

However, men, children and senior can all develop a yeast imbalance and its accompanying symptoms. Superficial yeast infection symptoms cause the development of a white substance in the mouth (where it is known as "thrush") or a cottage-cheese textured substance discharged from the vagina. When the white substance is present on the tongue, it does not wipe away easily, and when it is wiped off, it may leave red, irritated tissue below, or it may even bleed.

A yeast infection on the skin may result in flaky, itchy, burning patches or raised bumps. It is also commonly found in the finger- or toenails, which will cause the nail to lift from the nail bed.

In recent years, yeast infections have increased and some experts believe that it is mutating and becoming resistant to anti-fungal medications, especially *Candida glabrata*, which is the second most common yeast pathogen in people that causes irritation similar to Candida albicans. Once treated, Candida albicans is often followed by an infection of Candida glabrata, scientists are finding.

Some health practitioners believe that internal yeast can cause a multitude of serious symptoms that include constant fatigue, stomach bloating, abdominal pain, indigestion, severe weight fluctuations due to the yeast feasting on the sugar in your blood. This may actually cause you to crave sugar even more and result in dips in energy.

Yeast infections can also lead to urinary infections, vision problems, hair loss and itchy, irritated skin. Other symptoms may include a chronic runny nose, depression, frequent illnesses, mental fogginess and a loss of interest in sexual activity.

Yeast infections are typically diagnosed by the doctor simply looking at your symptoms. If he or she is unsure, then a bit of the white substance will be scraped off and examining it under a microscope.

Some anti-fungal medications and lifestyle and diet changes may control Candida levels in the body and ease the symptoms. However, once the drug treatment stops or the diet efforts wane, the yeast, which has simply gone dormant while you've attacked it, and its uncomfortable symptoms may return, so diligence is necessary in keeping you healthy and symptom-free.

Chapter 2: What Causes Yeast Infection?

As mentioned, yeast infections are caused by the loss of friendly bacteria in the body that fights off the overgrowth of Candida that always exists in the body, but usually in small amounts. Once out of balance, the Candida fungus, which was harmless in moderate levels, overtakes the friendly bacteria and runs amok, creating yeast infection symptoms like a white coating on the tongue, white discharge from the vagina or inflamed, itchy rashes anywhere on the skin.

This process of overwhelming yeast growing within the body can be caused by a variety of factors, such as taking certain medications or coming into contact with someone who has a yeast infection (through bodily fluid or airborne Candida spores). Many people with compromised immune systems, such as those with cancer, diabetes or AIDS or who are hospitalized for chronic illnesses or surgery, are at a higher risk of developing a yeast infection.

You can contract a yeast infection through exchanging fluids with another person, such as through sharing food, kissing or intercourse. Babies can sometimes get a yeast infection from their mothers through breast feeding and being in close proximity.

Very often, if you take certain antibiotics to stave off a medical condition, it will likely kill off the friendly flora bacteria in your body that keep Candida under control. The Candida overtakes the remaining bacteria and grows out of control. If your immune system is not strong enough to fight back against the Candida, you will wind up with a yeast infection of varying degrees, depending on the strength of your immune system.

Poor hygiene and habits can also cause yeast infections to grow, such as allowing sweat to linger in the folds of the skin, not wiping properly after using the restroom, wearing too-tight underwear and being exposed to some chemicals (such as fabric cleaners or perfumed feminine products) that can cause an allergic reaction that eventually leads to a yeast infection.

Infections in Women

It is estimated that 70 percent or more women will have a yeast infection in their lives, and more than half will have recurring yeast infections. Candida is particularly rampant in women because it feeds off progesterone. In fact, women often experience a flair up during their periods when progesterone levels naturally increase.

Yeast infections in women may also be triggered by lack of sleep, stress, eating lots of sugar (which the Candida also loves to eat), overall poor eating habits, illness, taking antibiotics or birth control pills and even pregnancy. While a yeast infection can be transmitted during intercourse, it is not considered a sexually transmitted disease, and it's more likely you will get a yeast infection from the other causes, although you and your partner can certainly pass an infection back and forth through sex.

Recent research discovered that a woman's ovulation cycle can actually put her at greater risk for contracting infections such as Candida albicans and sexually transmitted diseases. A woman's immunity naturally dips during ovulation to allow for sperm to survive and for an egg to be fertilized, and this vulnerability can be an optimal opportunity for yeast to infect her body.

Infections in Men

While women suffer from yeast infections more often, men can certainly get them, too. And they can be present on any area of the skin, including the penis, which is particularly uncomfortable. Like women, yeast infections in men are caused by an imbalance of Candida and the bacteria that typically fights it off.

Men can also develop an infection if they have a poor diet, are stressed or have a low white blood cell count. Some condoms that contain the spermicide nonoxynol-9 may actually cause Candida to grow more rapidly. However, practicing safe sex with a partner who may have a yeast infection is important to stop the cycle of passing it back and forth to one another.

Infections in Children

Because yeast naturally exists in the mother's vagina, babies may contract a yeast infection during birth. Also, babies often develop yeast infections in their mouths, which can be transferred to their hands if they suck their thumbs—and babies can pass the infection to their mother's nipple if they are breastfed. Because moisture is trapped in diapers, a yeast infection can grow in this area for babies, too, causing irritation. Antibiotic use among children is another major cause of yeast infections, as well.

Infections in Seniors

With age, yeast infections can be more common, and this is caused by weakened immune systems, the slowing down of cell regeneration and higher levels of toxins in the body. Surgery and other medical treatments can create an opening or yeast to grow in vulnerable areas. Dentures can cause oral thrush in seniors and those with type 2 diabetes may also be more susceptible because their blood sugar is already compromised, and the yeast will fester in this environment. Stress, poor diet, hormone replacement therapy and failing health can also cause yeast infections to recur in seniors.

Unfortunately, some seniors who are bed-ridden or immobile in nursing homes often suffer from yeast infections that can grow in the folds of the skin that are not taken care of cleaned properly.

Chapter 3: Yeast Vaginitis

Candida albicans is the most common type of yeast infection and it affects nearly two-thirds of all women during their lifetimes. Because yeast naturally occurs in the body and an overgrowth happens easily, it can be difficult to control, but not impossible.

The yeast can be introduced into the vagina through sexual intercourse, or the yeast that already exists there can increase through the use of antibiotics, which kill off the protective bacteria that control the amount of yeast in the body. It is believed that diabetes, pregnancy or use of oral contraceptives (birth control pills) can trigger a vaginal yeast infection, also called *monilial vaginitis*. A poor diet with a lot of sugar and carbohydrate consumption also creates an ideal environment for yeast to grow.

The vagina is particularly susceptible to yeast growth due to the moist skin, which the yeast thrives in (as well as other folds of the skin and the mouth). When present, a yeast infection in the vagina causes a burning sensation, itching, pain during sexual intercourse or urination and on-going soreness as well as a discharge of a white substance that has a cottage-cheese-like texture. Although this discharge is not always present in yeast infections, it is the leading indicator for doctors to make a diagnosis of a yeast infection.

When suffering a yeast infection, a woman may experience non-stop discomfort for up to about two weeks, which can really affect her mood, cause extreme embarrassment and even lead to depression. The burning and itching can constantly demand her attention and significantly reduce her quality of life while she is suffering.

A proper diagnosis with a pelvic exam is necessary. The doctor will look for cracks in the skin or small white bumps as well as discharge. If discharge is present, it will be examined under a microscope to make a positive identification. This is necessary since some other vaginal irritants (such as herpes or gonorrhea) can cause similar symptoms, and left unchecked, a yeast infection can continue to grow inside a woman's body and cause more serious, even life-threatening, situations.

At-home Care

Many over-the-counter anti-fungal products are available at drug stores without a doctor's prescription to ease the symptoms of a yeast infection when taken properly and for the entire recommended duration (usually three to seven days). These include creams and suppositories.

However, these treatments should only be used if you are quite sure that you are suffering from a yeast infection (it's not your first) and not another problem. Most women who have recurring yeast infections are well aware of their symptoms. If this includes you and your symptoms are not severe and you're not pregnant, using an over-the-counter treatment can be an inexpensive and efficient way to clear up your yeast infection.

You should also practice other good habits at home, such as wiping from the front to back after using the restroom; wearing loose-fitting cotton underwear (no synthetic fabrics like polyester, nylon or lycra); wearing cotton underwear underneath pantyhose; cleaning well after sexual intercourse and eating yogurt regularly due to its high content of active cultures that promote the growth of good bacteria that can help to fight off yeast growth.

You may also want to avoid using perfumed feminine hygiene products that can cause an allergic reaction. And wear loose clothing that doesn't constrict your body. Since vaginal yeast infections can often occur around the time of your period, using pads instead of tampons are a good option, since tampons can restrict the infection within your body. Also, be sure to change your pads frequently to avoid excess moisture next to your skin.

While douching may seem like a good way to keep you clean, it can actually strip away the good bacteria and other helpful secretions and allow the yeast to grow, so douching should be avoided if a yeast infection is present.

If sex during this time is painful, consider using a lubricant and always have your partner wear a condom so he will not be infected by the yeast. Also, some women have found that avoiding baths during a yeast infection and taking showers instead helps to eradicate the irritation more quickly.

Seeking Medical Help

If your infection is severe or if you simply want to clear up an infection without at-home creams, your doctor may prescribe a medication such as diflucan or nizoral, which you will take orally. You will take diflucan just once, but nizoral may need to be taken twice a day for up to two weeks. However, these oral medications may have side effects such as stomach pain, nausea and headaches, so your doctor may recommend that you use a cream or suppository instead—particularly if you are pregnant.

You will want to contact your doctor for an exam if you have not had a yeast infection before, if you are not sure what it is, if symptoms don't improve with over-the-counter products or if it gets worse. A yeast infection that doesn't respond to treatment may actually be a sign of HIV, so you need to be examined.

A study by St. Louis University found that as many as three out of four women took it upon themselves to self-diagnose and treat themselves for a yeast infection. However, many times, the woman didn't, in fact, have a yeast infection. Treating a non-yeast infection with treatments geared for yeast infections can make the actual problem worse, so seeing a doctor for a definitive diagnosis is critical in getting the proper care. The actual issue may be inflammation, dry skin or a sexual transmitted disease—all of which require a different treatment than anti-fungal medication.

Recent research has shown that, among healthy women, the microbes in the vagina can vary to a large degree, so your doctor may customize your treatment plan. So some women may have a certain microbe make up that would typically be considered harmful, but, in fact, are normal for them.

Some women (an estimated 5 percent) suffer from recurrent vulvovaginal candidiasis (RVVC) and have four or more vaginal yeast infections in a one-year period. These are women who often have diabetes or issues with their immune system and may need more intensive anti-fungal medical treatment and restrictive diets to keep their yeast under control (see chapter 8).

Prevention

In addition to regularly practicing the good hygiene listed above, you can make some changes to ensure your yeast infection does not return. Wear loose clothing and underwear with cotton crotches and do your best to keep your vaginal area clear of excess moisture (such as from sweat or wearing a wet bathing suit for extended periods of time). If you suspect your sexual partner has a yeast infection (see chapter 5), be sure that he is examined and treated, or you may pass the infection back and forth to one another without relief.

Diet-wise, begin to eliminate excessive sugar consumption such as desserts, sugary juices, soda and candy. You may also want to cut back on yeast-products, like carbohydrates and starchy foods. Instead, consume a cup of yogurt a day, which is rich in friendly bacteria that will keep yeast at bay in your digestive tract. Since yeast infections are also associated with obesity, you may want to explore options for losing excess weight through diet and exercise.

Be sure you keep your stress levels in check and get adequate sleep every day, as stress and poor sleep habits are also linked to an increase in yeast infection outbreaks.

Chapter 4: Yeast Infection on Nails

You can develop a yeast infection anywhere on your body, but especially those areas that come into contact with moisture regularly—such as your hands—thanks to the micro-organism Candida albicans. Yeast spores also travel easily between body parts. In fact, babies often transfer thrush (a yeast infection in the mouth) to their hands when sucking their fingers. However, yeast infections to the finger or toenails more often occur among adults over age 60 who have diabetes or a weakened immune system, have hangnails or ingrown toenails or live and/or work in a hot, humid climate.

People who wash their hands excessively or work in conditions where their hands are often wet (such as cooks or dishwashers) are more susceptible to developing yeast infections on their hands—typically within the nail beds. Moisture can get trapped between the nail and the skin, which is the ideal condition for yeast to grow and infect the skin. Use of antibiotics can also cause an excess of yeast growth under your nails, as it often does in other areas of the body. (The affliction actually occurs to the skin, not the nail itself, although the nail will appear to react.)

Known as *yeast onychomycosis*, this infection can happen under your toenails, too, especially if you use communal showers (like at the gym) or a public swimming pool. Speaking of the gym, if you work out a lot and have sweat trapped in your socks and shoes, you are at greater risk for developing a yeast infection in your toenails. You may notice that your toenails are turning yellow or brown or have grown thicker in texture.

If you have a yeast infection in your nails, you may start to notice your nails growing more brittle and breaking more easily. You may see color changes, including yellow, white or green areas around your nails as the infection starts to take hold. The naturally glossy texture of your nails may start to dull as well, and you may even notice some pus oozing from your nail.

Left to fester, the yeast infection will eventually destroy your nails and cause them to lift away from the nail bed, crumble along the edges, collect debris beneath them or even fall off. The skin below will likely be swollen, tender and scaly. If your nail stays in place, it may feel swollen, particularly around the cuticle area, and sensitive to touch. If the nail falls off, it can take up to a year to grow a new one, however it will likely be absent of the infection.

Many ailments can cause changes in your nails, such as ringworm, aging, injury, hormonal changes, psoriasis or other bacterial infections, so a definitive diagnosis with a doctor is important. A yeast infection in your nails may be harder to determine than yeast infections in other areas of the body, due to the fact that nails can be affected by so many other issues. Your doctor will likely take a sample of your nail by either cutting a bit off or drilling a sample out. It will be sent to the lab for testing and diagnosis.

Self Care

Although washing your hands regularly is a good way to keep illness away, excessive washing can allow moisture to seep under the skin, so you may want to cut back on how often you wash your hands, especially if you have been diagnosed with a yeast infection. If you feel the need to clean, opt for a non-soap cleansing gel from time to time.

You will also want to keep your nails well-trimmed, and your doctor may even suggest shaving it back quite a bit so that moisture cannot find its way under the nail bed. Do not overly trim your cuticles because an injury will invite yeast to collect. Some believe that yeast does not like an acidic environment, so soaking your nails in vinegar may help to kill off the yeast, although this hasn't been scientifically proven.

Medical Treatment

If you have diabetes or are experiencing nail pain along with other yeast infection symptoms, it's definitely time to see a doctor. Since creams and lotions are not well absorbed into the nails (although they may offer you some instantaneous—albeit temporary— relief), your doctor will likely prescribe an oral medication that can take up to a year to take full effect. The common oral medications include fluconazole, itraconazole and terbinafine.

Like other medications, these carry some side effects and can interact with other medications, so their use will be closely monitored. (Some of the medications have been linked to liver problems.) Your doctor may try some of the newer treatments for yeast infections in the nails, such as light therapy, topical treatments with electrical currents to help them absorb and a new nail lacquer, ciclopirox, which has shown some promise in resolving nail yeast infections.

Prevention

Nail infections return about half of the time. The No. 1 way to avoid a recurring nail yeast infection is to keep your hands and feet clean and as dry as possible. Keep your feet clean and dry them well—including between your toes. Avoid walking in public showers or gyms barefoot (bring a pair of flip-flops) and stay out of public pools. Remove sweaty socks as soon as possible and avoid wearing shoes that are too constricting. Some believe that acrylic nails smother your natural nails and can cause a yeast infection to fester under your nails.

Do not share your towels, nail clippers of other tools you use to maintain your finger or toenails. When getting professional manicure, bring your own sterilized tools and avoid using those that the manicurist has used on other clients. When washing dishes or gardening, wear vinyl gloves, but do not let water settle in the fingers of the gloves. Smoking has also been linked to an increase in yeast infections in the nails—so take the necessary steps to quit. Do not bite your fingernails.

Chapter 5: Yeast Infection on Penis

Unfortunately, yeast infections are not just for women. Men can certainly get them, too. Although it is not terribly common, women who are infected with a yeast infection can pass it on to their male partner through sexual intercourse. Because yeast prefers to live in dark, moist areas, it is more prevalent in women's genitalia than in men. However, yeast will infect men and cause uncomfortable, embarrassing symptoms, particularly for men who are uncircumcised.

Candida balanitis is the scientific name for a yeast infection on a man's penis. It can cause an inflamed rash or patches of skin that appear red or white and itch and burn at the tip of the penis for a week or longer. Som men experience an odor or a white discharge as well, and can also develop small white bumps on the top of their penis. It can spread throughout the man's crotch and include the inner thighs, scrotum and even the buttocks. The penis, however, will experience the greatest pain since it contains many more nerve endings than other body parts.

Like other people at risk for yeast infection, men who take antibiotics, have weakened immune systems, HIV, diabetes, poor dietary habits, obesity or other illnesses, are more susceptible of contracting a yeast infection on their genitalia or elsewhere.

A male yeast infection may have similar symptoms as jock itch, but the causes are different. Jock itch is a fungal infection as well, and is caused by excessive sweating (typically among men who work out a lot) or when sweat is trapped in the folds of the skin on a person who is obese. Instead of candida, however, the fungus that causes jock itch is called dermatophytes, which acts similarly to yeast infections and can be transferred through sexual contact.

At-home Treatment

Men can use an over-the-counter cream (like Monistat) to treat a yeast infection, too. It may take twice-a-day applications for a week or so to clear up. However, if it is the first infection, it should be looked at by a physician first to ensure it is not something else, as yeast infections in men can often be confused with herpes, and vice versa.

It is best for both partners to be treated and to abstain from sex if symptoms have developed until the yeast infection has cleared up in both people. If you decided to have sex, you may both find it painful and the man should wear a condom to protect his sensitive skin and to avoid passing the infection to his partner. Lubrication may help to make the experience more comfortable for both people.

Also, be sure to wash your genitals and your hands after having sex. However, sex is not the only cause for yeast infections for either the man or woman, so it is not considered a tradition sexually transmitted disease.

Lifestyle habits such as stress reduction and immune-boosting nutritional choices (like more fresh fruit and vegetables) and eating probiotic yogurt regularly can help a man to overcome a yeast infection and even keep another episode at bay. For diabetics, it's imperative to keep your blood sugar under control and avoid eating lots of starchy or sugary foods. A clean diet will help to keep yeast under control.

When choosing condoms, read the ingredient list and avoid any that contain the spermicide nonoxynol-9, which has been shown to increase yeast growth in men up to four times as much as those without the ingredient. Choosing a condom without spermicide will allow you to avoid that risk.

Also, wear loose-fitting cotton underwear to keep you more comfortable while you get the infection under control. Ditch your tight jeans and opt for workout clothing that is made with cotton instead of spandex, which does not breathe well and can lock in moisture.

Don't linger in a wet bathing suit and generally keep yourself clean and dry as much as possible, yet use natural soaps to avoid allergic reactions to fragrant or chemically laden soaps.

Medical Help

If needed, men with be treated with the same oral anti-fungal medication that women are given, primarily diflucan and nizoral.

However, the first may cause allergic reactions, and the second will destroy all of the bacteria and can even interfere with testosterone production. You may also be monitored to ensure the medications are not causing a problem with your liver, which they've been known to do.

Chapter 6: Yeast Infection in Mouth

A yeast infection in the mouth is typically known as "thrush." Like other forms of yeast infections, it is caused by an over production of yeast that prefers to grow in dark, moist areas on the body—like the mouth.

Like other areas, yeast is normally present in the mouth. Good bacteria keep it in check and stop it from overgrowing into an infection. However, when that balance is disturbed, through excess stress, taking antibiotics or suffering from an illness, yeast cells can multiply quickly.

An infection of thrush can cause a white coating on the tongue that does not wipe away easily. It may also cause redness that is sore in the mouth, as well as cracks along the sides of the lips. The coating and small lesions or bumps can spread to the upper mouth, cheeks, tonsils and all the way back into your esopha-gus.

Thrush makes swallowing difficult or painful and people with advanced forms of thrush often experience a feeling that food is stuck in their throat. Thrush victims may also experience fevers as the infection deepens.

Your doctor will often be able to simply look at your mouth and determine if you are suffering from thrush. When he or she wipes away the white coating, it will reveal irritated, red skin below that is sensitive and may even bleed. If needed, the scrapping will be sent to the lab to confirm the diagnosis.

If your doctor is concerned that thrush has spread to your esophagus, you may need a throat culture or x-ray to confirm it. People with weakened immune systems may find that the thrush spread more quickly to other organs in the body.

In young babies (under two months old) thrush is quite common and looks like milk curd on the insides of their cheeks, lips and tongue. The baby may come into contact with the yeast that naturally occurs in its mother's birth canal. Also, if a breastfeeding mother is taking antibiotics, it can cause a bacteria imbalance in the body that allows the yeast to grow into an infection.

As in adults, when thrush is wiped away from a baby's mouth, it will reveal red, irritated skin that might bleed. It will likely be painful and the baby may cry when trying to breast feed or being fed a bottle. It's vital to keep any items going in the baby's mouth very clean, such as bottle nipples or pacifiers.

As the baby gets older and stronger, he or she will develop a stronger immune system that will fight off the thrush. In other words, the baby may simply outgrow it. To ease symptoms, the doctor will likely provide a topical medicine that can be rubbed on the affected areas of the baby's mouth. This will likely clear it up within a week, but a stronger medication may be prescribed in more serious cases. Any family members who have yeast infections should be treated, as yeast spores can travel through the air or by touch and can be easily transmitted to a baby.

Smokers may be at higher risk for contracting thrush due to the fact that smoking cigarettes adds chemicals into the mouth that can throw off the balance of micro-organism in the mouth.

Dentures that are not fitted properly can also create gaps between the gums and the dentures where yeast will be right at home and flourish. Many older people who wear dentures also suffer from dry mouth syndrome, which also disrupts the mouth's chemistry and allows the yeast to grow into an infection.

At-home Treatments

Digestion of sugars start in your mouth, so eating large volumes of them come in direct contact with the yeast wreaking havoc there. Start to cut out sugary foods like cookies and ice cream, and cut back on foods that include yeast, such as beer and bread.

If you are breastfeeding and experience a yeast infection due to your baby's thrush, be sure to keep your nipples clean and dry and wear disposable nursing pads in your bra, so they yeast spores don't transfer to your clothing.

If you wear dentures, remove them at night and clean them well by soaking them in a denture cleaner. Rinse them well in the morning before putting them on again.

To relieve pain associated with thrush, choose cool foods that are easy to swallow like ice cream or jell-o. Cold liquids like water or iced tea may also soothe your mouth. You can also rinse your mouth with warm salt water a few times a day. Cranberry juice may also ease the infection.

Seeking Medical Help

Your physician or dentist may prescribe you medications to ease the amount of yeast in your mouth, including oral or liquid medication or lozenges. You will take these anti-fungal medications for up to two weeks. Because thrush can often be present in the event of other medical maladies, your physician may want to do a thorough workup to determine its cause and any underlying health issues you may be having.

If your doctor prescribes you an antibiotic and you are concerned about an impending yeast infection due to the medication, ask him for a prescription for a strong probiotic, or increase the amount of yogurt with live cultures that you're consuming.

Prevention

Good oral hygiene is a must, and that includes brushing and flossing twice a day. However, you'll want to avoid mouthwash because it can kill off the good micro-organisms in your mouth. You should be visiting your dentist a few times a year anyway, but if you have recurring yeast infections in your mouth, you may want to see your dentist more often. If you smoke, find a way to stop.

You may also want to avoid certain foods that have been shown to trigger a thrush outbreak, such as dairy foods, foods that contain yeast, MSG, pickles and foods that have been smoked, like fish or meat.

Chapter 7: Systemic or Internal Yeast Infection

While the causes of systemic or internal yeast infections are the same as those that occur on the skin, the symptoms can be quite different. Like other forms of yeast infections, an internal episode occurs when the friendly bacteria in your intestines is overrun by yeast that has been allowed to grow excessively. This can be caused by taking antibiotics, corticosteroids or birth control pills. This type of infection can fester inside your body and occasionally appear externally as an itchy, painful rash on your skin.

It may also occur in people who have poor nutritional habits, consume too much sugar or have diabetes or food allergies. For those with weakened immune systems, being exposed to environmental toxins or pollutions can trigger an internal yeast infection.

A gut that is yeast-friendly is typically found in people who eat a lot of refined carbohydrates and unhealthy fats, but have too few servings of dietary fiber. People who have internal yeast infections find that they begin to crave sugary food due to the fact the yeast is feasting on the current supply of sugar in the blood.

This type of deep yeast infection can manifest anywhere on the skin, but especially in areas where moisture can get trapped, such as under the breasts, in the arm pits or even on the face or scalp. People who are obese and have excessive folds in their skin may also develop irritating rashes in these areas. This type of yeast infection also does not discriminate based on gender—anyone can get it.

Those who have had surgery or had medical devices inserted into their bodies (such as catheters) are at an increased risk of developing an internal yeast infection due to the opportunity the surgery or insertion has opened in the body. Health practitioners should do their utmost to ensure a completely sterile environment when treated patients to avoid allowing this type of infection to take hold.

Yeast infections can live on the surface of the skin or in the intestines, and people who have recurring yeast infections likely suffer from the deeper internal version.

A food allergy, such as milk or wheat, can cause internal damage, and the yeast will find a home in the lining of the stomach or intestines. People with this sort of yeast infection may find that they experience stomach discomfort and bloating when the yeast causes the food to ferment instead being digested. This further fuels the sugar and carbohydrate cravings.

Left untreated, yeast can linger in the internal systems of the body and lead to more serious conditions such as chronic fatigue syndrome, Crohn's disease, fibromyalgia and other autoimmune diseases. These types of conditions often cause chronic pain and a severe lack of energy that can be traced back to an excess of yeast within the body. Other symptoms may include constipation, mental fogginess, acne, depression, memory problems, indigestion, lack of sex drive and nasal inflammation.

A stool sample is typically necessary to make a diagnosis of internal yeast infection, in order to test the levels of yeast and other micro-organisms. A simple blood test will also reveal of excess of yeast, as will a throat culture.

Systemic infections may require a tissue sample and biopsy to expose the Candida. When caught early, systemic infections can be treated with oral medications, but if severe, the patient may need to be hospitalized to ensure it is completely eradicated.

Left unchecked, yeast can burrow its way through the lining of the intestines, leading to a medical issue called "leaky gut syndrome." Leaky gut syndrome occur when the intestinal lining has been damaged and undigested food and certain bacteria "leak" into the blood stream.

If the yeast ventures into the blood stream, it can poison it (a condition called sepsis)—which is considered a life-threatening incident. In fact, nearly half of the people who have this sort of serious yeast infection will die from it. Yeast infections can also find their way to the brain, which can cause a severe change in mental ability and behavior.

Testing for and treating an internal yeast infection is generally quick and inexpensive, and certainly not worth the risk of letting it linger. People with weakened immune systems, AIDS, diabetes or who have undergone chemotherapy should be particularly watchful for the signs of internal yeast infections, which their bodies will have a difficult time fending off.

Medical Help and Prevention

Hospitalization may be necessary if the patient begins to have fever and/or nausea with their other yeast infection symptoms. A bout of thrush may require a hospital stay and intensive medical treatment, but skin infections can likely be treated with medication or at-home treatments without needing to be hospitalized. However, those with compromised immune systems may need medication through an IV in order to fend off the invading yeast.

Some anti-fungal drugs that your doctor will prescribe will attack and damage the yeast's cell wall and cause the yeast to die. Those medications include miconazole, tioconazole and others that typically end in "-azole."

A complete dietary overhaul may be suggested in addition to anti-fungal medical in-

tervention to stop the yeast from growing out
of control again.

Chapter 8: Treatment Options & How to Stop Yeast Infections from Coming Back

The key to treating a yeast infection is to restore the balance of good bacteria and a harmless level of yeast in the body. To do that, many medications are used to ease symptoms and target the yeast cells to kill them off. Some natural supplements and holistic treatments are believed to help reduce the amount of yeast within the body or on the skin.

Significant and stringent dietary changes can also help to restore balance within the body and keep the yeast from returning. However, once the medication is discontinued or the diet efforts are not maintained, yeast—and its nasty effects—can return. Reacting quickly to the symptoms can stop it in its tracks and slow the infection's progression and the damage it can do.

Traditional Treatments

If you are suffering from what you suspect is your first yeast infection—or if you are unsure what the problem is—it's vital to go to your physician for an accurate diagnosis. If your yeast infection is isolated to your genital region, your doctor will likely recommend a topical treatment that you can buy over-the-counter at the drug store. These are typically applied before bed every day for a week or more, but be sure to read all of the instructions and use the treatment until your infection is completely gone. Those treatments include:

- **Miconazole (Monistat)** is an over-the-counter topical cream that is used to treat vaginal infections, and can also be applied to the penis in the event of yeast infections. This medication may also be available in suppository form, which is inserted into the vagina.

- **Clotrimazole (Lotrimin)** can be purchased over-the-counter in topical creams to treat yeast infections on the skin. This may also be available as a suppository, which some people prefer because they are less messy and come in stronger doses, so they need to be used for fewer days.

- **Butoconazole (Gynezol, Femstat)** is another cream that is inserted in the vagina. You should not have sex while using this cream because it can break down the latex in condoms.

- **Tioconazole (Vagistat)** is another nighttime cream used to treat vaginal yeast infections. When using this or any other vaginal medications, be sure to wash your hands thoroughly after applying.

If your yeast infection is more severe, your physician may prescribe you a medication that is either injected or taken orally. Like the majority of prescription drugs, these may be effective in controlling yeast, but have certain side effects you should be aware of before you take them. The typical medications for a yeast infection include:

- **Flucytosine (Ancobon)** is a prescription anti-fungal medication that is taken orally. It may cause problems with the blood or play a role in kidney or liver disease. It may also cause your sun to be more sensitive to sunlight.

- **Fluconazole (Diflucan)** is a prescription medication that's taken orally or intravenously to treat serious cases of yeast infections. It may cause allergic reactions and interact with other medications. It needs to be used with caution, as it may increase the risk of heart or liver problems and can cause some digestive problems with sugar or dairy.

- **Ketoconazole (Nizoral)** can come in oral or topical form and is effective in treating serious fungal infections, such as yeast, athlete's foot or ringworm. This prescription medication may worsen liver disease or cause an imbalance of stomach acid.

- **Clotrimazole (Mycelex Troche)** is available through a prescription in lozenges to help combat yeast in oral thrush.

- **Itraconazole (Sporanox)** is available in capsules through a doctor's prescription. It is used in serious cases of yeast infections of the mouth, throat and esophagus as well as the finger or toe-nails. It kills the yeast and prevents its return.

In the case of an internal or systemic yeast infection that is threatening your overall health, you doctor may hospitalize you until it is under control. You will likely receive anti-fungal medications intravenously to stop the yeast from invading other internal organs.

Natural/Holistic Treatments

Due to the cost of side effects of certain medications, some people prefer to seek holis-tic treatments that they can purchase in health food stores.

You'll likely want to take more than one of these natural supplements to quickly combat the yeast in your system. Be aware that some supplements can interact with other medica-tions you may be taking. Speaking with your physician or a holistic expert can help you to eliminate any unwanted interactions or exces-sive doses of these supplements. Here are some supplements that have shown to be par-ticularly beneficial in killing yeast:

- **Probiotic supplements.** While you can get probiotics through foods like yogurt, your physician or holistic health practitioner may suggest supplementing your diet with probiotic tablets to help rebuild the amount of friendly bacteria in your stomach and intestines, which will work to eliminate the overactive yeast.

- **Fatty acids.** Found in many foods, oils (like olive and coconut oils) and supplements, these have been shown to kill off candida albicans.

- **Easily digestible multivitamin.** This will help with your overall health, since many people who suffer from yeast infections are typically missing essential nutrients in their diets.

- **Black walnut husk.** Juglone, the active ingredient in black walnut, has been shown to be an effective anti-fungal agent. You can find the extract in supplement form or included as an ingredient in candida supplement remedies.

- **Garlic.** This is a proven natural anti-fungal agent that can quickly kill off excess yeast, and it also contains anti-inflammatory properties and boosts overall health. You can eat a clove or two of fresh garlic daily or take up to 900 mg of garlic supplements a day. Keep in mind, however, that garlic has a blood-thinning effect, so your doctor may want to ensure that it doesn't interfere with other medications you may be taking.

- **Goldenseal.** The alkaloid berberine is the active ingredient in goldenseal, and it is an anti-fungal that has been found to be effective in improving digestive issues and wound healing. It's available in capsule or liquid form, but be sure to start with the lowest dose recommended on the packaging, as goldenseal can be bothersome to the liver if taken in large quantities.

- **Cat's claw.** This herb is known to help improve your immune system and white blood cell count, which is important when fighting off a yeast infection. Follow the bottle recommendations for taking cat's claw capsules, which usually recommend one to two 1 gram capsules three times a day. Pregnant women should avoid cat's claw. Also, be aware that cat's claw has blood thinning properties.

- **Caprylic acid.** Found in coconut oil, this acid is a powerful anti-fungal that kills yeast cells. It's especially effective when combined with other anti-fungals, such as grapefruit seed extract, garlic and oregano oil. You can either consume a few tablespoons of coconut oil daily or take caprylic acid in 600 mg capsules.

- **Oregano oil.** This is a powerful anti-fungal supplement because candida will not build up a resistance to it as it does with other anti-fungal treatments. Also, oregano oil contains antivirals and antibiotics that help the body to recover, as well as anti-inflammatory properties to assist in maintaining good health. You can take oregano oil in liquid form by adding a few drops to water twice a day. Or take soft gel tabs twice a day.

Home Remedies

You may find relief of the itching and discomfort of a yeast infection by applying certain home remedies, such as:

- Apply plain, sugar-free yogurt to your genitals until the symptoms subside. Then rinse off and dry your skin. Some have found relief by coating a tampon with the yogurt and inserting it inside your vagina.

- Insert a garlic clove or an all-natural garlic gel tab into your vagina. Garlic kills yeast quickly. You can also take garlic supplements to reduce the yeast from the inside out.

- Vinegar has been touted as a yeast killer, but you do not want to apply it directly to your skin, as it will be quite painful. Instead, add a few drops to your topical vaginal yeast medication. Some people suggest adding vinegar to your bath water, but taking a bath may cause your yeast infection to linger. Instead, add some vinegar to water and rinse your genitals with the mixture. Dry your skin completely.

- Applying Mediterranean oregano oil to affected skin, including the penis, may improve a yeast infection because it attacks the center of the yeast cell, which causes it to die. Be sure to dilute oregano oil with another oil (such as olive oil) because it can burn the skin when used at full strength.

- If you suffer from thrush, rinse your mouth regularly with warm salt water to ease symptoms and drink cold water throughout the day. Avoid sugary drinks.

- Soaking finger or toenails in a mixture of apple cider vinegar and water is an effective way to clear up a mild nail infection. Soak them for 20 minutes twice a day. Applying tea tree oil mixed with olive oil may also help to eradicate the infection.

- If a regular toothpaste is too painful on mouth sores, make your own with baking soda and water while your mouth is healing. You can pour a bit of baking soda into your hand and mix in enough water to create a paste. Rinse with warm water. Be sure to buy a new toothbrush once your infection has healed.

• For babies suffering from yeast infections in the diaper area, make a rinse of warm water and apple cider vinegar and apply it to the affected area. Allow it to dry before putting on a diaper. Plain, sugar-free yogurt can also be applied topically and will treat and soothe the infection. You may also want to crumble a flavorless garlic tablet into your baby's food to help clear up the infection internally.

Lifestyle Changes

There are many steps you can take to make sure your yeast infection goes away and doesn't come back. Here are the main habits you need to change or adopt:

• Stay dry. Because the yeast grows in moist areas on the skin, be sure to fully dry the skin between your toes, under your breasts, under your arms, between your fingers, on your buttocks and under your scrotum. Also, do not sit around in a wet bathing suit or sweaty workout clothes. Change into dry clothes as soon as possible and be sure to wash your swimsuit between each wearing.

- Wear pads. During your period, use pads instead of tampons during a yeast infection so that the tampon doesn't hold the infection inside of you.

- Loosen up. Do not wear underwear or pants that are tight. Now is not the time for you tight jeans or spandex workout clothing. Opt for natural fabric, like cotton, for your underwear. Or at a minimum, find panties and pantyhose that have a cotton lining.

- Manage sugar. If you have diabetes, it is likely that you also have suffered from yeast infections. Be sure to closely monitor your blood sugar levels, as a drastic change can hint to a yeast infection as the Candida loves to feed off of the sugar in your blood.

- Lose weight. People who are over-weight or obese tend to had excess folds in their skin. Yeast loves these warm folds, especially if they are moist with sweat.

- Reduce stress. Not only will excess stress tempt you to eat un-healthfully, it is also been found to play a role in al-lowing a yeast infection to grow in strength. Take care of yourself, find ways to relax and delegate chores and errands that stress you out.

- Sleep well. This is necessary for your immune system to stay strong, which is important in fighting off any infection, including a yeast infection. Good sleep habits include keeping to a regular schedule, sleeping in a dark room, avoiding television before sleeping and cutting back on caffeinated drinks early in the day.

- Stay clean. The yeast will be happy if you do not pay attention to the moist areas of your skin. Always practice good hygiene and clean yourself well after sexual encounters. Also, if you're using a vaginal cream to combat your yeast infection, be sure to clean your hands well after applying it. When washing your clothes, use a hotter temperature of water and try adding a cup of white vinegar during the rinse cycle.

- Avoid irritating chemicals. Fragrances or other harsh chemicals added to feminine cleansing products and perfumes can highly irritate your infection by causing an allergic reaction. This is true of scented bath soaps, bubble bath and scented tampons and pads. Also, buy plain white toilet paper as the inks in printed versions can also be irritating.

- Don't douche. Your body is built to naturally cleanse itself, and douching can clear away helpful bacteria during this process. Also, after using the restroom, be sure to wipe yourself from front to back to avoid bacteria from entering your vagina.

- Keep your hands and feet clean and dry. Yeast loves to borrow under your nails and infect the nail bed, but you can keep it at bay by wearing gloves to do household chores and be sure to remove sweaty or wet shoes and socks. Also, choose shoes that fit properly and are not too tight.

- Consider changing your birth control. Oral birth control has been associated with an increased risk of recurring yeast infections as are certain condoms that include spermicide. You may want to switch to a diaphragm, plain condoms or an intrauterine device (IUD). Also, chose water-based lubricants instead of petroleum-based lubricants.

- Keep your distance. If you're suffering from a yeast infection, avoid kissing and sexual intercourse for the sake of your partner. Plus, if he or she gets the infection, it can be passed back to you. Yeast spores aren't limited to the skin. They can take flight by air and infect others.

- If you must take an antibiotic for another illness, you may want to take precautionary measures to ensure the antibiotic doesn't incite a yeast infection, which they are known to do. Consider taking a probiotic supplement while on your antibiotic or eat a cup of yogurt a day during the course of your treatment.

- Help babies to avoid a yeast infection by keeping the diaper area clean and dry. Sprinkling some talcum powder will help to keep baby's skin dry. Allow your baby to go diaper-free from time to time, and if needed, use a protective cream. To prevent oral thrush in babies, be sure to keep all bottle nipples and pacifiers clean and try to keep the baby's fingers out of his mouth by covering them with thin mittens.

Diet and Nutrition

Because yeast will grow when given the nutrients that it feeds on, your diet may hold the key to keeping yeast infections at bay for the long term. Many books and articles have been written about the right diet to follow. The challenge is that cutting out the necessary food items will cause feelings of "withdrawal" as the toxins leave your body. Remember that this feeling is temporary, and after about 10 days, it will ease and you'll be feeling much better and will have come a long way in reducing the yeast in your body.

Here are the key foods to eat, avoid and incorporate into your daily diet. Keep in mind that if have recurring yeast infections and you veer too far from this diet, the yeast and your symptoms will return. Get back on track to tamp down yeast growth. You may be able to occasionally enjoy a sugary or carbohydrate treat in moderation.

Foods to Eat

Wholesome foods like fresh fruit and vegetables.

These are essential for overall health, but most fresh produce also contains inflammation-fighting nutrients that will help your body recover and fight off the yeast. Aim for a wide variety of fruits and vegetables in a multitude of colors to get the most nutritional value. The best vegetables include:

- Broccoli
- Kale
- Spinach
- Tomatoes
- Peppers
- Green beans
- Bok choy
- Peas
- All types of lettuce
- Zucchini
- Galic
- Ginger
- Onions
- Eggplant

Fiber.

Eating more fresh fruits and veggies will help with this, and you may even want to try a fiber supplement to help your digestive process work more efficiently while your intestines are healing from the damage the yeast has done. Plus, you'll simply feel better.

Yogurt.

Opt for plain, unsweetened yogurt so that you will not be unwittingly consuming more sugar. The active cultures and probiotics in yogurt will help to promote the growth of friendly bacteria that will get the yeast back under control.

Fresh meats and proteins.

Beef, chicken, turkey and eggs are sugar-free and will help to satiate your hunger and improve your overall strength. You can eat nuts, which are a decent source of protein as well as omega-3 fatty acids, but they can contain mold that you don't want to consume. Simply wipe off nuts with a clean paper towel before you eat them and choose raw, natural versions instead of roasted and salted versions.

Seafood.

Many of these contain omega-3 fatty acids, which are essential in overall health. Aim for a couple servings per week.

Whole, yeast-free grains.

Opt for yeast-free options to get lots of healthy fiber that will improve your digestive function and remove toxins from your body. Stay away from white bread. Here are some of the best choices:

- Oatmeal
- Quinoa
- Buckwheat
- Barley
- Brown Rice
- Millet
- Spelt
- Couscous

Herbs.

Some of these, particularly garlic and oregano, are strong yeast killers. Plus they reduce inflammation and relieve constipation. Plus you can add flavor to your food without unhealthy salt.

Oils.

Coconut and olive oils are particularly helpful in killing off yeast.

Tea.

No matter if you choose green, chamomile, peppermint, lemongrass or any other type of tea, they all contain anti-fungal properties. You can gargle with basil tea to relieve thrust and a rosemary tea may ease symptoms when applied topically.

Foods to Avoid

Sugar.

This may be particularly difficult because the yeast in your body is devouring the sugar in your blood and making you crave sugar even more. Nevertheless, you will want to take whatever measures necessary to keep your sugar intake to a minimum so that you will eventually starve the yeast cells.

Sugary juices.

Since yeast feeds off of sugar, these can be a somewhat unlikely source of extra sugar in your diet. As you wean yourself off of juices, you may want to try to dilute them with half juice and half water. Try to work towards reaching for plain water to quench your thirst.

Beer and other alcohol.

Since it is made with yeast, it's best to avoid beer so that you do not add more yeast to your body that is already overactive with it. The same holds true for other alcohol, which contains sugar.

Packaged/processed foods.

These items, such as potato chips, bagged cookies and desserts, frozen meals, bottled salad dressings and others, are stripped of their nutrients and quite often, sugar and preservatives are added. Packaged/processed foods and sugar have been shown to increase inflammation, which is the opposite of what you need to do while you are fighting off a yeast infection.

Yeast-enhancing fruits and vegetables.

While most fresh produce is helpful to achieve optimal nutrition, some may inspire more yeast growth. Stay away from fruits like dates, figs, grapes, prunes and raisins, in particular. The majority of vegetables are OK, with the exception of mushrooms (which are a type of fungus), olives and starchy options such as potatoes, beans, parsnips and squash.

Sweet condiments.

For now, you'll want to skip items like honey, maple syrup, agave nectar, relish, ketchup and cocoa. You can, however, have carob.

Processed meats.

Lunch meats, bacon, hot dogs and sausage contain nitrates that have been shown to be unhealthy and lead to conditions like cancer and heart disease. They are also difficult to di-gest—especially if you are suffering from an intestinal yeast infection.

A Sample Diet

For the first seven or so days, you will want to eliminate all toxic-building food items and focus on detoxifying foods, such as vege-table soup that includes onions, celery, and greens. You can add potatoes and carrots to the soup while it is cooking, but remove them before consuming the soup so you'll avoid the carbohydrates.

You may also want to add a detoxifying drink made with soluble fiber and water or olive oil and garlic. You may be able to find pre-mixed detox drinks at health food stores.

After your detox, you will want to stick to yeast-fighting foods, and avoid yeast-producing foods. Combine fresh vegetables with every meal, along with low-fat, quality protein (fish, raw nuts, yogurt) and complex carbohydrates that are fiber-rich, such as brown rice, buckwheat, oats or quinoa.

Breakfast:

Try eggs, hot oatmeal or whole-grain bagel with nut butter. You can also try a smoothie made with soy milk and whey powder.

Lunch:

Have a fresh vegetable salad or a vegetable soup. Add some quality protein or a sandwich made on yeast-free bread.

Dinner:

Same as lunch, focusing on quality protein and fresh vegetables.

Snacks:

Chew fresh vegetables or nuts (except peanuts), rice cakes or have a plain, sugar-free yogurt with chopped fresh fruit, such as berries.

Beverages:

Water should be your go-to beverage, but you can also have herbal teas, which are strong anti-fungal. Soy milk is a good option to add some protein and vegetable broth can quench your thirst without the sugary mindfield found in sodas or fruit juices.

Chapter 9: Recipes for a Yeast-free Diet

With a few simple substitutions, you can still enjoy your favorite foods. You may need to swap out regular milk for coconut milk and use quinoa flour in bread recipes, but you'll avoid adding yeast to your body while it tries to fight off the infection. If you find you need extra sweetness to your foods, you can use sugar substitutes in moderation. However, some experts believe that because these artificial sweeteners are so much sweeter than regular sugar, your body may crave more sweetness. So be sure to use them in very limited amounts.

Quinoa hotcakes

Ingredients:

- 1/3 cup quinoa flour
- 2 eggs
- 1 teaspoon coconut oil

Instructions:

Mix all ingredients until well blended and spoon onto a hot griddle. Avoid using syrup. Add some chopped berries to add a bit of sweetness.

Yogurt parfait

Ingredients:

- 1 cup sugar-free plain yogurt
- 3/4 cup fresh berries
- 1/2 cup nuts, like walnuts

Instructions:

Layer yogurt, berries and nuts in a tall glass until you have used all of the ingredients.

Chocolate-banana smoothie

Ingredients:

- 1 cup coconut or other nut milk
- 1 medium banana
- 6 cacao beans, raw

Instructions:

Place all ingredients in a blender and mix until smooth. To make it frostier, add a cup or two of ice.

Hummus

Ingredients:

- 2 cans garbanzo beans (drain one can, but keep the liquid in the other)
- 1/4 cup sesame seeds
- 1 tablespoon olive oil
- 1/4 cup lemon juice (fresh is preferred)
- 1 teaspoon cumin
- 1-2 cloves of fresh garlic

Instructions:

Place all ingredients in a food processor and blend until smooth. Serve with fresh vegetables or slices of yeast-free bread.

Yeast-free flat bread

Ingredients:

- 1 teaspoon olive oil
- 1-1/2 cups distilled water
- Sea salt
- 1 cup whole-grain flour
- 1 cup unbleached white flour
- 1/2 teaspoon non-aluminum baking powder

Instructions:

Mix olive oil, water and a dash of sea salt followed by the flours and baking powder. Mix until the batter is smooth. Heat a skillet to medium heat and add the batter, ensuring that it coats the entire bottom of the pan. Cook for about a minute or until the top begins to dry, then flip and cook the other side.

Tuna salad

Ingredients:

- 1 package flake tuna
- 1/2 yellow onion
- 1/2 teaspoon olive oil

Instructions:

Mix tuna, onion and olive oil in a bowl and add any herbs for extra taste. Smear on wholegrain, non-yeast bread.

Onion soup

Ingredients:

- 6 onions of your choice
- 3 teaspoons olive oil
- 4-5 garlic cloves, grated

Instructions:

Thinly slice and stir fry onions in olive oil over medium heat. Add garlic and cook for a few minutes longer. Add sea salt and other herbs of your choice to season. Add enough water to cover onions and garlic and allow to simmer for 30 minutes before eating.

Yeast-free pizza dough

Ingredients:

- 2 cups flour
- 1 teaspoon salt
- 2 teaspoons baking powder
- 2/3 cups water
- Vegetable oil

Instructions:

Mix and knead together everything except the oil. Do not overwork the dough. Spread onto pizza pan and use a brush to cover lightly with vegetable oil. Top with your favorite toppings, including sugar-free tomato sauce, shredded cheese, Italian herbs, ground pork or hamburger and lots of vegetables. Bake for 15 to 20 minutes at 425 degrees.

Chicken and vegetable stew

Ingredients:

- 1 tablespoon olive oil
- 2 chicken breasts, skinless, chopped in-to bite-size pieces
- 1 potato, peeled and cut into one-inch pieces
- 1 onion, diced
- 1 cup celery, diced
- 1 tomato, chopped
- Salt and pepper

Instructions:

Heat oil and sauté chicken in a large pot until cooked through. Add all vegetables and enough water to cover all of the ingredients. Reduce heat to a simmer and cook for an hour. You may need to add more water throughout the hour. Add salt and pepper to season. If you're concerned about the starch in the pota-toes, remove them before you eat the stew.

Yeast-free custard

Ingredients:

- 2 cups milk
- 10 drops artificial sweetener drops, like Stevia
- 3 eggs
- 1 teaspoon vanilla extract
- 1/8 teaspoon sea salt
- 1/8 teaspoon nutmeg

Instructions:

Heat milk and sweetener until it just begins to boil. Cool for 10 minutes. In a bowl, beat the eggs, vanilla, salt and nutmeg until smooth. Add milk slowly and mix well. Divide mixture into four ramekins. Place ramekins in a roasting pan filled with water and bake uncovered at 325 degrees for 50 to 60 minutes until cooked through. Chill in refrigerator before serving.

Conclusion

Now that you have a better understanding of where your yeast infection stems from, it's time to get it under control once and for all and stop it from coming back. Keep in mind that the first and most important element is to determine if you are, indeed, suffering from a yeast infection.

While taking charge of your health is important, misdiagnosing yourself and using a yeast infection medication could lead to further problems. Also, if your problem is something else (herpes or other sexually transmitted diseases are often confused with a yeast infection), those medical conditions will go untreated and can eventually lead to more serious problems.

Once your doctor has determined that you are suffering from overactive Candida, be sure to maintain your medical treatment and follow up with the dietary and lifestyle changes outlined in this report in order to keep the yeast from returning.

If you suffer from a recurring bout of yeast infection, remember to attack it early before it leads to a more serious infection that can threaten your health. As you can see from this report, you do not have to spend a lot of money, and you can create many soothing treatments with ingredients you own in your kitchen. Plus, with a few smart food swaps, you can clear out your diet to keep the yeast away for the long term.

While yeast infections are particularly unpleasant, it is reassuring to know that you can take an immediate and active role in your recovery.

Appendix: Glossary

AIDS: Acquired immune deficiency syndrome, the final stage of the HIV infection and disease. People with AIDS are more susceptible to developing yeast infections because their immune systems are weakened, so they are not as able to fight off the infection.

Antibiotics: These are medications that are prescribed to kill micro-organisms in the body. Although they are meant to attack unfavorable organisms, the sometimes also kill good bacteria that keeps yeast from growing into an infection. Taking antibiotics is considered one of the main risk factors for yeast infections.

Candida: A genus of yeast. There are about 20 different types in the human body, a few of which lead to bothersome yeast infections.

Candida albicans: The most common type of yeast fungus in the body that causes yeast infections in the genitals, mouth, skin and other areas.

Candida balanitis: A yeast infection on the penis.

Candida glabrata: Previously known as torulopsis glabrata, this type of yeast was not typically considered troublesome until the past decade or so. When candida alicans is eradicated, candida glabrata often takes over.

Candidiasis: A yeast infection caused by any of the forms of candida.

Ciclopirox: A Food and Drug Administration-approved nail lacquer that is used topically to eliminate a yeast fungal infection on the finger or toenails.

Dermatophytes: A type of fungus that causes jock itch, which is sometimes confused for a yeast infection in men.

Diflucan: A fluconazole injected medication that is used to treat fungal infections in the mouth, throat, esophagus and other internal organs, such as the abdomen, lungs and blood.

Leaky gut syndrome: A medical condition that occurs when the lining of the stomach or intestines is damaged and undigested food and bacteria are "leaked" into the blood stream. Yeast infections that grow through the intestinal walls are believed to cause leaky gut syndrome.

Miconazole: An over-the-counter vaginal cream used to treat yeast infections.

Monilial vaginitis: A yeast infection in the vagina that is most commonly caused by candida albicans.

Nizoral: A topical cream that is used to treat yeast infections on the skin.

Nonoxynol-9: A spermicide often used in condoms that is associated with increased growth of yeast infections in men.

Probiotics: "Friendly" bacteria that can be found in foods like yogurt, these are considered healthful and able to help control the levels of yeast within the body.

Recurrent vulvovaginal candidiasis (RVVC): Suffering from a vaginal yeast infection four or more times within a year.

Thrush: A yeast infection in the mouth that effects the inner cheeks, tongue, roof of the mouth and esophagus.

Yeast: Micro-organisms in the fungi family, which are generally considered harmless and live naturally in the human body. They become dangerous when conditions occur that allow them to grow in numbers and develop into an infection.

Yeast onychomycosis: A yeast infection in the finger or toenails and nail beds.

25355257R00055

Printed in Great Britain
by Amazon